"In his writing, Josephs provides a wealth of information and support which will benefit many stroke survivors and their families. Each chapter is a stand-alone piece covering very important topics related to stroke. Survivors who have the book will be able to return to it to receive support and information at any time."
Pat Kasell, Manager
COURAGE STROKE NETWORK

"A book written by a stroke survivor who vividly shares his personal experiences and that of other stroke survivors. The information, suggestions and motivational messages will prove invaluable to new stroke survivors, their families, friends and the professionals who are instrumental on their road ahead to recovery."
Thelma Edwards, R.N., Director of Program Development
NATIONAL STROKE ASSOCIATION

In "Stroke: An Owner's Manual," Arthur Josephs transcends the typical roles of patient and even "survivor" to become an articulate and inspiring spokesperson on Life after a stroke. As a writer and former litigating attorney, who experienced a stroke more than 10 years ago, Josephs is both a participant in his own recommendations and an expert witness, providing invaluable insights and information to fellow survivors, as well as to health care providers, who take the time to inform themselves on the inner experience of stroke.

In this new era of patient advocacy, consumer rights, and what the federal government calls "participatory actions research," Josephs' guide stands out as a pioneering work with an empowering message. I can only hope that Mr. Josephs' efforts to do more than merely survive his encounter with stroke will inspire others living with a disability or chronic illness to share their stories. The rapidly expanding field of medical rehabilitation needs to be broadened and enriched by the contributions of knowledgeable "consumers" like Mr. Arthur Josephs.
Margaret L. Campbell, Ph.D.
MEDICAL SOCIOLOGIST and
CO-PRINCIPAL INVESTIGATOR for the
"COMPARATIVE STUDY of AGING and DISABILITY"
RANCHO LOS AMIGOS MEDICAL CENTER

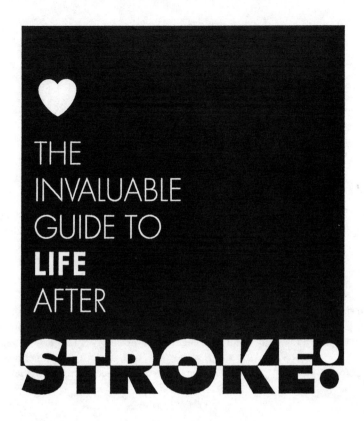

THE INVALUABLE GUIDE TO **LIFE** AFTER

STROKE:

AN OWNER'S MANUAL

By Arthur Josephs*

*Someone who's been there

STROKE: AN OWNER'S MANUAL

by Arthur Josephs

The Invaluable Guide to Life After Stroke

Published by:AMADEUS PRESS
Post Office Box 13011
Long Beach, C.A. 90803 U.S.A.

Copyright 1992 by Arthur Josephs
Second Printing 1993
Library of Congress Catalog Card Number:
91-77440

Publisher's Cataloging in Publication
(Prepared by Quality Books Inc.)
Josephs, Arthur, 1929-
    Stroke:an owner's manual:the invaluable guide to life after
stroke/ by Arthur Josephs
    p. cm.
    ISBN 0-9631493-9-3

    1. Cerebrovascular disease--Patients--Guide-books. 2.
Cerebrovascular disease--Patients--Rehabilitation--Popular works.
I. Title. II, Title: Guide to life after stroke.
RC388.5.J6 1992   616.81
                                          QBI92-307

With love to Shirle, the one person who has given meaning to my life and my words.

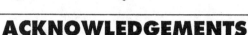

ACKNOWLEDGEMENTS

For the friendship, encouragment, knowledge, constructive criticism and gentle strokes which made this book on stroke possible, I wish to thank Norman Corwin, John Hermann, Marianne Simpson, Doctor Stuart Mann, Doctor Margaret L. Campbell, Thelma Edwards, Pat Kasell, Millie Selenkow, Mary Buck, my son Gregg and my three favorite daughters, Stacey, Randi and Amy. For showing me the doorway to self-publishing and then pulling me through it, thanks to Charles Edward Sherman and Trudy Devine.

♥

TABLE OF CONTENTS

Stroke: An Owner's Manual

♥

FOREWORD

by Doctor Stuart H. Mann
Fellow, Stroke Council, American Heart Association

Physicians are usually preoccupied with the physical aspects of stroke and frequently fail to appreciate the emotional, personal and family aspects of this disorder. The author, an attorney, brings to light his own experience, as well as those of patients with whom he has come in contact at various support groups. A long journey back to health for himself is described with great feeling and compassion.

The author realizes that both his style of living and his personality have changed since his stroke. That fact is also readily recognized by his family, friends and colleagues. The main experience was the need to assume responsibility for his own healing process and to learn to cope with his disability. All of the Stroke Team have a place in the recovery process, and this includes the physician, as well as the physical, occupational and speech therapist. In the author's case, the speech therapist was of major help in treating not only about functional speech, but helping with the cognitive dysfunction that often accompanies a stroke. The Stroke Team alone is not sufficient and for a significant recovery to occur it takes motivation and persistent work by the stroke survivor for there to be meaningful improvement.

I am excited that STROKE: AN OWNER'S MANUAL is now available to stroke survivors and their families. It is indeed a self-help resource and an information guide for stroke survivors, their families and care-givers. Stroke does not respect any age, sex, or race and it usually strikes when most unexpected.

As a neurologist interested in stroke, I particularly enjoyed the chapter on seizures. Few people realize, including physicians, that seizures are a common sequelae of stroke. There is a need to explain this condition to both the patient and the family so that they can be prepared for this rather frightening event. The author has described his seizures specifically and the condition in general in a detailed and understandable way.

The difference between damage to the left hemisphere of the brain versus the right hemisphere of the brain is also discussed in an interesting and detailed manner. There are so many different types of stroke, depending on location and cause, that it is useful to have it discussed in a way that patient and family can understand.

STROKE: AN OWNER'S MANUAL will become a supportive companion to stroke survivors and their families as they attempt to rebuild their lives. At last, we are finally giving stroke the attention that it deserves in a manner which can be easily understood. It helps the stroke survivor adjusting to the illness by obtaining insight and knowledge about the condition. The author has retired from the practice of law and has turned to another occupation, which is writing. Two of his plays have been produced and he writes several columns for local publication. This is his first attempt at a book, and is a fine example of the type of work that can be performed by a stroke survivor.

Stroke: An Owner's Manual

♥

INTRODUCTION

T hursday was the day when I headed out to the golf course, placed all the stress of being an attorney inside a white golf ball, put the ball on a tee, and tried to hit it out of sight. My three friends who made up the regular foursome usually laughed at the result—a hook, a slice or a roller. Golf "duffers" need to get off their duffs more than once a week if they hope for improvement.

But on occasion, even at age fifty-three, I could drive the ball 200 yards straight down the fairway. My only other exercise during the week was an occasional battle with weeds in our yard or some minor repair job around the house. "Anything you want me to bring back for dinner?" I called out to my wife, Shirle, as part of our routine. "Birdie, eagle?" "The usual," she answered. "You." It was January 28, 1982, our thirty-first anniversary. "But make it early. Beth and her latest will be dropping by to drink a toast. Your favorite daughter will expect you to be here, golf or no golf."

"I promise. I won't even stop for a beer with the guys."

Our four girls knew I referred to each one of them as my favorite, but Beth, the youngest, would be extremely upset if I missed meeting the man of her dreams. I didn't make it home for dinner until two months later. I had a stroke.

My family and I knew nothing about strokes. Our lack of knowledge caused the two month hospital stay to be a living hell for all of us. The following months were even more agonizing. The stroke damage forced me into instant retirement. Shirle faced not only the economic worries but the peculiar behavior of a stranger in her home. If we knew then what we have come to learn over the years, a great deal of emotional distress might have been avoided. I felt compelled to become informed and try to assist other stroke survivors. Gaining experience for the writing of this manual has helped to turn my life around. The reading of this manual may help you start getting control over yours.

What survivors don't need to know before a stroke fills scores of medical volumes; what is essential for them to know after a stroke is the subject matter of this manual. The information and advice will help them maintain balance and, yes, even sanity, in the hours immediately following a stroke, the early days after release from the hospital, the years of recovery and the remainder of their stroke-influenced lives.

Most of my information comes from involvement with several stroke support and activity groups. Some is attributable to research undertaken to learn as much as I could about the stroke-induced changes in my emotions, personality and physical condition. Perhaps the greatest incentive to the research came from a speech therapist who upon being told of the location of my stroke lesion told me the following: I talk too much, act in ways which are socially inappropriate, have difficulty arriving at correct conclusions from a set of facts, fatigue easily, fight with my wife daily, can't balance a checkbook, and have trouble backing out of the garage. She was absolutely right, and I was determined to find out how she guessed so well. Of course, nothing she said was based on guess-work.

Every stroke is different and the ways they affect an individual are infinite. But there are common threads which run through the singular tapestries of illness created by dead brain cells. This work is a manual. It will help guide you through the darkness surrounding a terrifying disease. And, hopefully, it will replace terror with hope.

♥

PREFACE

You have suddenly been hurt in a terrible and mystifying way. You've lost some degree of control over communication, emotions or movement. There's a thought you want to express, but you can't speak; you see words on a printed page, but they don't make sense; someone speaks to you, but the sounds have no meaning. The tears won't stop. The rage won't stop. You strain to move a limb; nothing happens; one hand won't obey an order to open or close; some part of your vision is impaired ... and the list of afflictions goes on and on in unlimited shapes and forms of havoc.

But, you're lucky! Lucky to have survived, to have the opportunity to improve your condition. However, you won't realize that for some time. Some strokes are killers — the third leading cause of death in our nation. When the enormity of your loss hits home, you may wish you had died. Many of us felt the same way. Hang in there, the feeling will pass. In time you'll learn both the

21

bad and good news. The bad, that whatever loss you suffered may be permanent (stroke is a leading cause of disability); the good, that you will continue to get better for the rest of your life.

Several ground rules apply to what follows. For one, whenever the word "you" is used, it represents the person whose brain was damaged (stroke survivor, here- after often referred to by the single word "survivor"), or to the survivor's spouse, or any other person whose life is intertwined with him.

For another, though the masculine pronoun predomi- nates in references to the stroke survivor, that choice is arbitrary. Though the incidence of stroke is approxi- mately thirty percent higher in men, the damage inflicted by a stroke is equally devastating for a woman. They are also as successful as men in dealing with their strokes.

Finally, names have been altered, but the stories are true.

♥
Chapter 1

WHAT HAPPENED TO ME?

Comparison of stroke to heart attack.
Aphasia, right hemisphere damage, motor losses.

♥

Chapter 1

WHAT HAPPENED TO ME?

There are hundreds of thousands of stroke survivors each year. They are identical in two ways: each has lost a part of himself forever; each will improve in some degree for the rest of his life.

S troke. Most of us associate the word with an event which causes death of the elderly. Many believe the cause to be a vascular system so old it breaks down, resulting in some sort of massive internal brain hemorrhage. That may often be the case. But, though the risk of stroke increases with age, the aged have not staked out an exclusive claim to this killer. My circle of stroke survivor friends ranges in age from twenty-three to seventy-five, and there are reported cases of infants having strokes.

A cerebrovascular accident (CVA, stroke) is often referred to as a heart attack of the brain because each involves injury resulting from reduction of the flow of blood. However, while each may affect the survivor's health, strokes usually are cruelly disabling.

Many heart attacks occur because there is a cut-off of

blood supply to part of the heart muscle itself, causing an area of the heart to die. Survivors have less muscle tissue available to pump blood through the vascular system. Some strokes happen that way. An artery closes, cutting off a life-line of blood to brain cells. Strokes differ from heart attacks in that specific areas of brain cells perform specialized functions. Rather than having fewer cells to continue the activity, there may be none. Death of the cells means disturbance or loss of the function for which they were responsible.

The following examples have been selected from among those who suffered damage to the left brain hemisphere which processes language and symbols. Their losses are all the more tragic in a society like ours which places so much value on verbal communication.

Bill survived his stroke with no paralysis. He is able to talk, read and write; but if you speak to him, he can't understand a word you say. One tiny function of his communication system is destroyed .... those cells which "receive" spoken language. Sitting next to him in our support group meetings, I try to help him feel a part of the discussions by writing on a pad what is being said. No matter how fast I write, he is still a step or two behind in any discussion.

Another member of the group can understand what is spoken or written. He can formulate ideas in his mind, but whenever he tries to express himself, the only words he can say are a few numbers and several expletives. Another member is limited to the expletives. As an aside, almost every stroke survivor is able to curse regardless of the degree of damage to the speech center. It seems that expressing vulgarisms is a form of "automatic" speech which remains intact, and would seem to be appropriate in expressing the frustration resulting from inability to share one's thoughts.

A former teacher must struggle to verbalize a single word. Though she can think clearly, when she wishes to speak, the effort is gargantuan. The words in her speech center are upside-down and backwards! Unable to help, we watch her struggle as she mentally turns each word over and then around before being able to say it aloud.

Right hemisphere brain damage, on occasion, can cause problems with speech, but in a manner much different from those who get "locked out" of normal conversation. Most right brain injury induces an over-abundance of speech. At worst it produces nonsensical babbling, but the usual result is a person who simply talks incessantly. Joe combines two common results of damage in the right brain. He is unable to draw conclusions from a set of facts, and he talks too much. In other words, he goes on and on without ever arriving anywhere.

In too many cases language loss is accompanied by some motor loss. The severely hurt may be confined to a wheelchair. Paralysis usually affects one side of the body, such as a leg which needs bracing or a hand which is either tensed into an unusable claw or totally flaccid. As if all this pounding were not enough, motor losses are often aggravated by the added cruelty of partial blindness.

No two strokes are the same. Damage to persons in identical areas in the brain causes similar but different results. An analogy may be made to fingerprints. Though each of us has curved lines at the tips of our fingers, none of our prints are identical. Stroke rehabilitation specialists can analyze the type of dysfunction to be remedied, but each case has its own set of fingerprints.

With cell-life loss in the left hemisphere, the stroke survivor may have a problem with pronouns. He wants to refer to his friend, Jim, but in the process of reaching into the pronoun "grab-bag" of his speech center he may select "he" or "she" or "her" or "it" or "them." As a further complication, the choice is random, even in the same sentence. The pronoun selection disturbance usually is accompanied by an identical difficulty with numbers. Some survivors can't understand spoken language but can read. Some stroke survivors can read but can't write. Some survivors can read and write but can't form words well enough for them to be understood. Some survivors can form understandable words but need prompting in order to talk. These infinite differences have a sort of nightmarish quality. However, one thing is common to all stroke survivors. The road back to health is a never-ending tough struggle.

There are hundreds of thousands of stroke survivors each year. They are identical in two ways: each has lost a part of himself forever; each will improve in some degree for the rest of his life. For some fortunate ones, their cup will overflow; others will have to be content with teaspoons of success.

In our small group, we have witnessed the speechless talk; the motionless progress from wheelchairs to canes to unassisted walking; the confused discover clarity of thought; the deeply depressed, sweet joy; the lonely, love.

Stroke: An Owner's Manual

♥

Chapter 2

WHAT WAS IT THE DOCTOR SAID?

Insufficient medical advice.
Who can be trusted.
Doctors don't always predict correctly.
The road back to health.

♥
Chapter 2

WHAT WAS IT THE DOCTOR SAID?

Ordinarily, with time and care we expect to recover from sickness or harm. The cut heals, the bone mends, the fever breaks. Stroke survivors tell how they expected the damn thing to go away after a few weeks and how terrible it was to learn their loss was permanent.

Probably not much. Assuming, that is, your doctor is as busy as most people in the health care field. Sadly, due to the ever-increasing demands on the medical profession, many doctors who save lives have little time to tell patients all that they need to know about their strokes. Perhaps more significant is the fact that few survivors have any idea of what questions to ask the doctor. In some cases, the information received while in the hospital may not only be inadequate or incomprehensible, it may be very discouraging. Most doctors who treat the initial onslaught of a stroke are fighting to save a life. Once they win your war, they are immediately off to another battlefront. In trying to keep pace with today's onslaught of medically needy, doctors forget the healing quality from just a few words of encouragement, words which may turn nightmare into hope, and hope into health.

In the hours following the stroke I needed a powerful corticosteroid to reduce a life-threatening swelling in my head. I was alternately on a euphoric high or in a suicidal low. No one thought to advise my wife the drug might be the cause. She will never forget the terror to which she was needlessly subjected because she assumed it was the stroke which had caused my madness. I can assure you that I, too, would have done better during the weeks of my solitary horror if someone had gently taken my hand and whispered, "That drug may be the cause of your strange feelings. Hang in there. We'll take you off medication as soon as the swelling subsides."

A number of practitioners still tell patients not to expect any significant change after the first six months following a stroke. While optimum recovery from paralysis or numbness usually is reached within six months, that time limitation does not apply to everyone or every loss, for there are remarkable improvements among some stroke survivors long after six months. Speech and physical therapists won't state a time limit, because they're in the business of helping you get better for the rest of your life as long as you're willing to keep working. If nothing else, as long as you try, you can improve the quality of your life regardless of the amount of disability you may have suffered.

Bob, a witty, brilliant engineer, spent over three years in silence lying on a hospital bed. At first he could only communicate with his wife by blinking his eyes when, with a pointer, she selected the correct letter from an alphabet. After two years of non-oral communication, his speech therapist believed Bob could speak aloud if his weakened diaphragm got enough support to help power air from his lungs. He began to speak. A physical therapist believed Bob had enough movement in his chin to drive a specially designed electric wheelchair. He became mobile. When he isn't taking trips with his wife, he can be found wheeling about his neighborhood. Is six months the time limit for significant improvement from a stroke? Zipping by in his wheelchair, Bob would answer the question with a loud, verbal "Nuts!"

Vic, the patriarch of our group, had difficulty being understood because his stroke caused his speech to sound garbled. After years of therapy, he still required great effort to form understandable words. At age seventy-five, ten years after his stroke, an imaginative speech therapist had him place a twig in his mouth. Like Demosthenes who overcame a defect by speaking through stones, Vic began to talk with greater clarity. While there is no medical certainty the use of the twig caused the improvement, it is irrefutable that the man's fighting spirit brought him a measure of the contentment he dreamt about for many years. There was also paralysis to overcome. Through constant exercise, including swimming, he has reduced the limitation of movement in his right arm sufficiently to become a fierce opponent in a game of billiards.

Ordinarily, with time and care we expect to recover

from sickness or harm. The cut heals, the bone mends, the fever breaks. Stroke survivors tell how they expected the damn thing to go away after a few weeks and how terrible it was to learn their loss was permanent. Even years after the truth finally sinks in, most survivors fantasize they will awaken to find it was all a cruel nightmare.

You can't start too early on the long journey back to health. Most of us believe a person ought to be told at the outset that he's in for a hell of a battle and not to expect more than slow steady improvement. Nevertheless, for each person a time of mourning is not only proper but necessary. Each must grieve for that part of him which has died. The day will come when you will bury the fact that you aren't the person you once were. For most, the mourning lasts at least a year. During those funereal months, it takes a stout heart not to remain depressed. But the time arrives when you must end sorrow and start life anew. The sooner you can free your mind of the black mourning band, the sooner you'll take control of the real healing, that of learning how to cope with a disability. Chances are you'll discover you've become a better person. The success stories are too numerous to count. There isn't anyone who can't improve in some way through hard work and the desire to succeed, but you've got to be tough.

♥

Chapter **3**

WHY ME?

Causes of stroke.
Reducing the risks.
Examples of those who have overcome losses.

Stroke: An Owner's Manual

♥

Chapter 3

WHY ME?

If you "accentuate the positive" you may live a more healthy, high quality life. There's no place for guilt in a stroke survivor's fight to regain health and a new measure of self-esteem.

The sudden wrenching of a person from health to disfigurement and silence is so mind-boggling that many stroke survivors feel some sense of guilt, as if they somehow deserved to be punished. Poppycock. No-one "deserves" this nightmare. More importantly, there are solid, medically proven reasons for the affliction, causes which may be out of our hands. A stroke, although called a cerebrovascular accident, is no accident, nor is it somehow deserved. The longer you believe in the mumbo-jumbo of punishment, the less time you'll dedicate to taking control of your future health. The known risks which create conditions leading to a stroke are high blood pressure, smoking, high cholesterol, diabetes, chronic stress, obesity, heart illness, sedentary life style, oral contraceptives, aging, and a family history of vascular disease. You have the power to stay healthy by reducing some of these risks.

Some day when you and a medical practitioner friend have time, take a look at an angiogram of a brain. The complexity of arteries and veins will astound you. Hundreds of red lines intersect like threads of yarn tangled by a playful kitten. Since some of these conduits of blood in your brain are thinner than human hairs, it's easy for fatty tissue to build up in the artery walls and close an artery or to break off and lodge in a place where it blocks further blood flow. One of the astounding results of autopsies of soldiers who died in the Vietnam War was that a high percentage of very young Americans already had advanced cases of arteriosclerosis (thickening and hardening of the walls of an artery), while the Vietnamese had healthy arterial systems. The high fat diet of the Americans is considered partly to blame for the difference in vascular condition.

Sometimes, a crushing blow to the head will destroy these fragile, life-carrying arteries. Yes, you can add "trauma" to the many causes of stroke I've enumerated. One of my friends, a professor who rode a bicycle to campus, was not wearing his helmet when a collision with a car sent him airborne. He landed on his head. Though other parts of his body suffered only minor injuries, the brain trauma caused him to be without speech for over a year, and, sadly, after three years he is still without the full use of his limbs.

One member of our stroke support group was badly beaten about the head by a jealous rival. Although he had no motor loss, it took years of therapy to restore his speech. Now, after five years, he can talk without hesitation but his words are quite spare. "Genius," he'll say, not "He's a genius." Or, "Job couple bucks," instead of "The job pays me a couple of bucks." He had been an extremely successful salesman before the beating. Today, he does odd jobs for an old friend who is a major building contractor.

The most amazing survivor of the entire group was on an unswerving collision course with his stroke. He was overweight, diabetic, a three-pack-a-day smoker, a heart attack victim at age thirty-five and working in a stressful occupation. Few members of his family had been able to make it past the age of forty-five due to breakdowns in their arterial systems. He survived major combat wounds and two heart surgeries before an inevitable and terribly cruel stroke deprived him of speech and motion. He fought back from hospital bed to wheelchair to cane to leg brace to unassisted walking. His right arm and hand are as powerful as they once were, but he never attained his personal goal of being able to pick up a grain of rice with two fingers.

He worked equally hard to free himself from silence. His speech is restored, but labored. As if this were not enough, the threat of total closure of blood supply to his legs caused him to accept a surgical procedure which laid him open from stomach to knees for the insertion of plastic arteries. Forty pounds lighter and still sore from the surgical wounds, he began another comeback. Within two weeks of leaving the hospital, he mowed the lawns front and back. Some of us thought this was a crazy action on his part, but you've got to be a little bit "crazy" to have the courage to come back from where he's been.

A much loved member of the group has a great wit matched only by his dogged self-reliance and complete dedication to helping others. When he was a young boy, an infected left arm was amputated above the elbow. Nevertheless, at high school he lettered in football and baseball. Amazingly, he was a good batter with his one arm and played infield at the difficult position of short-stop. After catching the ball in his glove, he would toss it into the air, clamp the glove under his stump, then catch the descending ball with his bare hand to throw out the runner. Sadly, he followed in his father's footsteps which led him into local bars, and he had to spend years fighting the battle against booze. He beat alcoholism, too, and went on to become a popular disc jockey. However, his arterial system was so weakened by liquor it gave way, causing him to suffer a left-hemisphere stroke which deprived him of voice, profession and identity. He, too, fought to regain speech. As he is fond of saying, he knew he had graduated from speech therapy the day he was able to say Methodist Episcopalian because he considers himself to be an atheist. He learned to play one-armed golf and, although too old to letter in the sport, he's good enough to beat the average able-bodied player.

If any of the risk factors listed above apply to you or if any of the quick-sketch portraits of real people strike home, you may be able to answer the chapter title "Why Me?" How you choose to answer that question may help you to prevent another stroke. If you "accentuate the positive" you may live a more healthy, high quality life.

But remember these words of advice from those who have "been there." There's no place for guilt in a stroke survivor's fight to regain health and a new measure of self-esteem.

Stroke: An Owner's Manual

♥
Chapter **4**

DON'T LET IT COME AS A SURPRISE, BUT...

Depression, crying, fatigue, anger, selfishness, frustration, feeling cold, choking, sex.

♥

Chapter **4**

DON'T LET IT COME AS A SURPRISE, BUT...

Just as with the stroke itself, the more you know, the better chance you'll have to heal yourself.

In addition to the physical damage caused by the stroke itself, you may face other problems common to most survivors. These include depression, anger, selfishness, uncontrolled crying, fatigue, frustration, feeling cold, difficulty swallowing, and severely reduced sexual powers. Just as with the stroke itself, the more you know, the better chance you'll have to heal yourself.

DEPRESSION

You've had a sudden onslaught which may have stolen a part of voice or movement. Self-reliance, employment, self-control and independence are all gone. The fear of another crippling stroke rarely leaves. Isolation and loneliness are daily companions. The realization has set in that your body won't follow your commands, that whatever happened is permanent. Is it any wonder you feel deeply depressed?

You're not alone. Following a stroke, all survivors suffer some degree of emotional dejection. A few sink in darkness, never to find the light. Most conquer depression to go on to a new life. But the struggle is endless. Everyone I have met who successfully overcame his deep sense of loss needed assistance of some sort. There are three extremely valuable helpers, none of them "professional" in the usual sense of that word.

Time is the greatest healer. As the days turn to weeks, months and then years, there comes the realization you are free from danger. Time plus knowledge and the company of others who have fought the same fight will aid you in overcoming depression. A support group oriented towards education and the healing of the psyche will provide both the needed knowledge and the company. The collective experiences shared by members of that type of group adds up to a body of knowledge unavailable elsewhere. The friends you will meet are ones that will last for life.

Initially, educational and psychosocially oriented support groups are a must. Not only will you benefit from other survivors who will understand and help you get rid of your fears, but it's good to get out and be in touch with others. Don't let any difficulty you may have in communicating keep you from joining that kind of a group. So long as you can understand some of what others say, you will benefit. In time you will be aiding another, and so it goes. (See Chapter 18 for information on how to find a stroke support group or club).

Matt is unable to say a word, yet he is always the first

to sense that another is feeling low. Through body language and some rudimentary signing, he can lift that person's spirit. Once learning takes place and your self-esteem is restored, you may want to move on to a group which is focused on activities and socializing. The most likely sponsor of a group of that nature would be a local heart association. My personal theory is that surviving a life-threatening event like a stroke brings out the best or worst in a person. Those who are fighters find even greater reserves to carry on; the weak often falter until they fall by the wayside. In time the choice is yours alone, and it's a lonely one. You may not be able to command all body parts to work as they once did, but you can take command of your life.

ANGER, SELFISHNESS

The reasons stated above as causes for depression are just as likely to evoke anger and selfishness. Close family members need to understand these behavioral changes as much if not more than the survivor. Not only have unexpected burdens been thrust upon them, they are confronted by a demanding person who reacts with instant fury if ignored. After the onslaught of disabling illness and economic hardship, few relationships have any reserve left for such additional stress. Information, counseling and sharing available in family support groups can help smooth out the rough times.

49

UNCONTROLLED CRYING

You will cry a great deal. Don't blame feelings of depression. We all cry very easily, even years after the stroke. At the beginning, tears flow suddenly and without apparent cause, often stopping as quickly as they start. Be kind to yourself; don't feel ashamed. Doctors use the term "lability" to describe this condition. What they mean by the term is that a person's emotions have become unstable. I disagree. More likely the stroke has reduced your power to restrain emotion. Rather than losing stability you have gained heightened sensitivity. This gain applies especially to men. We are taught from early boyhood that crying is for girls. Grown men guard against showing tears because they think it's a sign of weakness. In some way the stroke destroys that guard. Tears flow easily. Be proud that you are in touch with your heart. Stroke survivors have a saying, "It takes a real man to cry." Sadly, so many real men learn the hard way.

The next time you go to a sentimental movie, take a seat near the front. As the lights come up, look back quickly and see how many men are dabbing their reddened eyes. They aren't stroke survivors but mere mortals able to let their feelings loose under cover of darkness.

Whether or not you feel shame, be assured there will be less and less crying as time goes on. Don't make the mistake of letting embarrassment cause you to isolate yourself from others. Tell your family and friends about the tears, then relax and be yourself. However, if you are

concerned about others who may frown upon men crying in public, let me suggest ways to help you regain
control. For one, change the subject of whatever conversation prompted the tears. For another, try to recall
something pleasant. These simple devices have worked
for many of us. Some, like Tony, refuse to forgive
themselves for the crying. His national heritage won't
allow him to believe that anyone except a sissy would cry
in public. Yet he faces a dilemma. His stroke changed
him from a hard-headed, non-caring, workaholic into a
gentle, loving person, constantly helping others. Both
joy and sadness bring tears to his eyes. Unable to
overcome his upbringing, he turns away or hides his face
when he expects tears. He refused to be nominated as
"Stroke Survivor of the Year" in our support group out of
fear he might cry when awarded the prize. We overcame
his disability. At the award banquet, the trophy was
handed to his wife.

FATIGUE

You will also fatigue very quickly. Those days of
constant activity from early morning to late evening are
over. A shoes off, hit-the-pillow for an hour nap will
become necessary at least once a day from now on.
Some stroke survivors need to nap several times. As you
merrily roll through the day, you will suddenly feel as if
someone let the air out of your tires. There may or may
not be a warning that it's time to turn out the light. Most
of us who can walk get a little wobbly or start to bump
into things. Even those who are not mobile get so

fatigued they must nap. Don't fight the sleep message being sent out by your brain. Get plenty of rest. However, you are not excused from regular exercise. Keeping physically fit strengthens the vascular system, lowers cholesterol and reduces stress—all helpful in minimizing the risk of another stroke.

FRUSTRATION

Expect to feel frustrated performing even simple tasks. Remember, you have received a tremendous blow to the brain. Your body won't necessarily operate on "automatic pilot" any longer. The best way to deal with the change is to take everything slow and easy. Do ordinary things at half speed. If you are able to operate a car, reduce your usual driving speed. You don't have the reaction time you once had. If you took small risks in traffic before, forget it. All risks are big now. The ladder you climbed with ease before is now a deadly menace. Let some other volunteer dry the dishes. Those with right hemisphere damage should expect difficulty trying to assemble things, especially according to written instructions. Most of all, be kind to yourself by accepting the fact there are limitations on what you can accomplish. Reduce your exposure to frustration. Be content with doing those things you still do well. Mac was an excellent artist until the stroke knocked out the use of his right hand. That loss is of little consequence when compared to his inability to speak. In the time he has learned to use non-verbal methods of communication, he has developed a somewhat slower but rather artistic left hand. Drawing on the right side of his brain, he is able to make regular cherished gifts of his creations to his friends.

FEELING COLD

Most stroke survivors usually feel colder than in the past. Whatever the reason, don't be surprised if you still want to wear flannel pajamas in summer, and need more than one extra blanket in winter. Also expect that the affected side of your body, left if the stroke was in the right brain and vice versa, may be slightly colder than the opposite side. The difference in sensation may feel strange, but it's nothing to worry about.

DIFFICULTY SWALLOWING

A post-stroke symptom which you must bear in mind when eating or drinking is that you may no longer be as adept at swallowing as before. It's easier to choke on food or get liquids into the windpipe. The answer? Cut smaller bites, chew the food thoroughly, drink and swallow smaller quantities.

SEX

Sex for survivors is not without its challenges and may yield some surprising advantages. The opportunities for lengthy foreplay and enhanced intimacy can be an unexpected boon for both men and women. Initially, there may be awkwardness at the physical level similar to that seen in a baby as it learns to walk, speak and cuddle. Discomfort and lessening of sensation can be turned into

into gain. Where previously a male's tendency to rush and focus on orgasm may have resulted in less gratification for his partner, a less hurried pace often results in a more lasting satisfaction for both lovers.

Massaging limbs, caressing, and the use of fingers can move the partner to arousal and create enhanced pleasure. Massage brings blood to muscles and tissue, thus adding substantial therapeutic benefit. Caressing, which in the passion of youth was often hurried, now becomes an end in itself. This is not to say that passion is diminished for the partner, merely that it is transformed into a more gradual, sustained expression of deeper intimacy.

For men, the ability to obtain and maintain an erection involves not only a delicate balance between the neurologic, vascular and hormonal systems of the body, but a mind free of great stress or anxiety. The man who suffers a stroke may have that delicate balance further shaken by the addition of hypesthesia (numbness) or the effect of medications required to prevent seizures or lower blood pressure. There is no way to calculate the devastation that sexual impotency can cause a male ego already battered by instant retirement and physical dependency. Nevertheless, here too, as with most stroke-induced losses, there are ways to regain a measure of self-worth.

Several procedures have been developed which can bestow artificial potency. Among these are injection therapy and the implantation of sophisticated devices to create an erection. I suggest that a doctor be consulted for detailed information.

♥

Chapter **5**

IF IT COMES AS A SURPRISE, A SEIZURE CAN BE FRIGHTENING

Seizures and their relationship to strokes.

♥

Chapter **5**

IF IT COMES AS A SURPRISE, A SEIZURE CAN BE FRIGHTENING

About 15% to 20% of stroke survivors will begin to have seizures within nine months to two years after a stroke.

Most people relate seizures to epilepsy. Few are aware of the fact that about 15% to 20% of stroke survivors will begin to have seizures within nine months to two years after a stroke. These seizures are rarely harmful and, most importantly, they are not forewarnings of another stroke. They occur because of the altered metabolism in the area where brain cells were destroyed. Without going into a technical discussion of the causes of such a seizure, it is enough to know the scarred area can bring on a type of electric storm which results in uncontrolled movements of all or part of the body, ranging from mild to very violent.

At times Hal's right hand thumb twitches. "This thing is crazy," he says, raising his hand for all to see. Though able to hold the thumb still, when he lets go, it begins quivering again. Seemingly with a mind of its own, his thumb relaxes just as abruptly as when it started moving.

Jim, who often has difficulty getting words out, experienced his first seizure at the worst possible time. He was swimming as therapy for his weak leg and paralyzed arm when the violent shaking began. Unable to shout "help" quickly enough, he started to sink below the surface of the water. Fortunately, a lifeguard at the pool spotted the problem and pulled him to safety. Jim had never been warned about the possibility of a seizure. Today, though he has been placed on medication which helps prevent further episodes, he has a decided preference for golfing.

My first seizure was the type usually classified as a grand mal. The electric storm crossed the mid-line of the two hemispheres of my brain, immediately knocking me out. I collapsed in front of my wife. Since we had not been forewarned, she thought I was having another stroke. Within seconds after their arrival the paramedics were able to stop my uncontrolled movements. I was able to recover my strength in three days, but my wife has yet to recover from the fright. To this very day the sound of a heavy object falling in our house strikes fear in her until she has assured herself of my well being.

Most of us who experience these episodes get a forewarning the seizure is about to happen. The warning, known as an "aura," usually takes the form of a strange sensation somewhere in the body. Mine is a queasiness in the stomach; George describes his as a buzzing in the head; Jim says he feels a chill across his chest. Those who experience auras usually have enough time to safeguard themselves from the threat of violent thrashing or unconsciousness. In whatever time your aura allows, find a space away from harmful objects, lie down on your side to keep your wind-pipe passage clear, try to relax without taking deep breaths. Hyperventilating increases the seizure potential. In this regard, recent experiments indicate some people have successfully prevented the onset of a seizure through the use of relaxation techniques. (Note: Some medical practitioners recommend lying on the back with something soft under the head because less harm may come from that position. They say lie on a side when the violence subsides).

Try to alert someone. Most seizures will stop in a few minutes, but if another begins after a moment of calm or if the seizure does not let up, paramedics must be contacted immediately. Continuous seizing can be life-threatening. It is medically imperative you report any seizure to your doctor. If any seizure causes unconsciousness, do not under any circumstances drive a vehicle until medically cleared to do so.

The good news is there are a variety of drugs which will substantially reduce the risk of re-occurrences. But the drugs cannot do the job alone. If you are seizure-prone, you must be careful not to bring about the altered metabolism which may trigger a seizure. When those of us who are at risk compare stories of what we did just before the seizure began, we talk of having had some alcoholic drink or being very stressed or failing to take our medication or getting excessively fatigued or being sleep-deprived or not eating regularly. An official with the National Epilepsy Society would add to the list of these triggering mechanisms the use of recreational drugs and the taking of certain over-the-counter medications. One head trauma specialist warns his patients away from saunas and hot-tubs because he believes the increase in body temperature is seizure-inducing.

The better news is that after three years from the date of the stroke, so long as you are careful to avoid the triggering mechanisms discussed above, the chances of having another seizure are substantially diminished.

The best news is that if you have not experienced a seizure within two years after the stroke, it is very unlikely you will ever have one. Hopefully, you will be among that eighty to eighty-five percent who don't have to face such a jolting surprise.

♥

Chapter **6**

HOME FROM THE HOSPITAL... NOW WHAT?

Location, type and cause of stroke.
Preventing the next one.

♥

Chapter 6

HOME FROM THE HOSPITAL... NOW WHAT?

If successful in your health program, you have as much chance to live on without another stroke as someone of similar age and background. Suffering one stroke does not mean you must suffer another one.

For you to survive, the doctors immediately had to discover the location, type and cause of your stroke. Knowing the location and type helped them decide if you needed immediate surgery (perhaps to clamp off a bleeding artery) or the use of drug therapy (perhaps to reduce a life-threatening swelling in the brain). Knowing the cause guided them in prescribing for your continued care whether by drugs (perhaps to thin blood, reduce high blood pressure, control diabetes) or by a change of lifestyle (perhaps to reduce stress or to eliminate smoking and drinking).

If you want to go beyond mere survival to live a meaningful life, you must do exactly what the doctors did: find the location, type and cause of your stroke.

Why location? Although the brain is still very much a mystery, the work particular brain areas perform has been thoroughly mapped. The stroke destroyed some of those cells, and though the injured area of the brain will heal, that healing will neither replace the lost cells nor bring them back to life. Thus, since each area of the brain performs a specific job, understanding the function which was damaged will help you to work around, adapt to, or try to overcome the loss.

As a simplified example of these options, consider having lost the function of one hand. You have always used both hands to tie shoelaces. You may "work around" the problem by wearing shoes needing no laces (velcro fasteners or slip-on); you may "adapt" by learning how to tie laces with one hand, or "try to overcome" the loss by using professional therapists to regain as much use of the hand as possible. Since motor losses are obvious, location becomes much more important in your understanding of any language disturbance (aphasia) you may have (usually a result of an injury located in the left side of the brain) or information processing disturbance which occurred (usually as a result of injury in the right side of the brain). Although each stroke is different, there are well-recognized general patterns.

Those people who have aphasia may suffer damage ranging from mere loss of clarity in verbalization to complete loss of communication. Many who are rendered speechless are fortunate enough to regain some verbal communication, sometimes as good as their pre-stroke speech. Restoration of verbal skills requires intensive work with professional speech therapists. Unfortunately, a few will never regain meaningful speech regardless of the amount of therapy. For them, communication must take place without words.

Severe damage in the right hemisphere can cause one to lose spatial contact with the left side of the body, babble words incessantly, and be unable to dress. Less severe damage causes behavioral changes so subtle they are generally accepted in our society as mere quirks. These include talking too much, behaving in socially inappropriate ways, having some difficulty with directions, being unable to balance a checkbook, misunderstanding another person's physical or verbal expressions, and reaching illogical conclusions from a set of facts. Nevertheless, these subtle changes may be catastrophic in close family relationships, especially when they are new to the stroke survivor's personality.

Damage to the cerebellum characteristically affects a person's balance and equilibrium. Sometimes the effect is so severe that unassisted walking isn't possible.

Why learn the cause and type of stroke? Stated bluntly, the knowledge, if acted upon, may help you prevent another one. Though having a stroke seems to be as sudden as being hit by a bolt of lightening, most strokes are the cumulation of many years of abuse of the vascular system. One of our group is fond of saying, "It took me a long time to get this stroke. I was fifty-three before it happened." Wouldn't it be comforting to know you may avoid the next bolt? To do so you must eliminate as many of the known risks of damage as you can control. If successful in your health program, you have as much chance to live on without another stroke as someone of similar age and background. In other words suffering one stroke does not mean you must suffer another one. The good news is that most of the risks can be reduced. Eliminate them and there may never be any more bad news.

Most of us oldtimers consider stroke survivors to be newborn babes until at least a year goes by. It usually takes that long to lose the paralyzing fear that another may occur at any moment. How painful to play a perpetual game of Russian-roulette; how comforting to have a hand in controlling your own destiny. Begin immediately to eliminate the risk of another stroke.

♥

Chapter 7

TAKING RESPONSIBILITY FOR YOUR OWN HEALTH

Research.
Other ways to take control.

♥

Chapter 7

TAKING RESPONSIBILITY FOR YOUR OWN HEALTH

So long as a person does not resign himself to defeat, there are victories to be won in the continuing battle to find a meaningful life after a stroke.

R égaining some control of your future begins when you realize you must be more concerned about your health than the doctor. Most people go through life never questioning "what the doctor orders." As mentioned earlier, however, since most doctors don't follow cases beyond the emergency stage, they may not be as accurate as therapists in predicting future improvement in a stroke survivor's condition.

Surprising? Not to members of our support group. A few uninformed practitioners still tell stroke patients that after six months from the date of a stroke no further improvement can be expected. As indicated earlier, such a statement is not only inaccurate, it may be extremely damaging. While it is true there are motor movements and some communication capabilities which may never be regained after the initial six month period, stroke survivors have been known to make progressive improvement in language skills for years. More importantly, there is no time limit for the development of strategies to compensate for losses. So long as a person does not resign himself to defeat, there are victories to be won in the continuing battle to find a meaningful life after a stroke.

Studies of the brain indicate that the uninjured hemisphere may have the ability to compensate for some losses which occur due to a stroke in the other hemisphere. For example, in a recent experiment conducted at California State University at Long Beach, stroke survivors who had regained their speech were asked to talk as an EEG measured their brain-wave activity. When healthy people speak, their left hemisphere virtually lights up during an EEG. However, in those who had to relearn speech, a greater than normal amount of right hemisphere activity occurred during their talking. This increased right side involvement was demonstrable proof the undamaged half of the brain was actively helping the injured half. If this increased activity represents one part of the brain "coming to the rescue" of the other part, might it not be a form of learning which will continue throughout life?

Regardless of whether or not the greatest amount of motor and language healing occurs during the first six months, we have witnessed many examples of a different type of healing which defies time—healing which takes the form of people compensating for and adjusting to an injury. How devastating it would be to give up trying because someone in white made a dark prediction.

Every motor-loss survivor is encouraged to strive for the time he is able to trade in the wheelchair for a walker, the walker for a cane, and finally the cane for unassisted walking. Every language loss survivor is encouraged to strive for the time he trades in verbal silence for other modes of communication. But the trade-off is hard work.

Evan didn't believe us when we said the day would come when he would no longer be imprisoned in a wheelchair. For months he suffered, for he had convinced himself there was no chance he would ever stand on his own two feet. Admittedly, he suffered one of the more damaging types of motor loss in his right limb. Most stroke survivors don't lose mobility in the shoulders or hips. The lower legs, arms and hands suffer the most. Evan couldn't command his right hip to move. Though the hip would support his weight, he could not take a normal step. About a year after the stroke, through expert physiotherapy, he learned how to take a step by swinging his entire right side. He's a free man again.

Rod, unable to speak, suffered the loneliness of the silent for several years following his stroke. He appeared to be somewhat fearful the first day he sat in on one of our sessions. For several weeks he responded to direct questions with no more than an embarrassed smile. After some imaginative and intensive speech therapy, Rod found his voice, adding approximately one new word a day to his speech vocabulary. He hasn't reached the stage of carrying on a conversation yet, but he's on his way. The embarrassed smile has given way to one of blushing accomplishment. Few doctors could have predicted such progress.

Many patients who are prescribed some form of drug therapy make no effort to be informed, placing complete trust in the doctor. We encourage stroke survivors to get answers to some basic questions: why the drug is needed; how it works inside the body; the side-effects it may have; whether other substances may interfere with its effectiveness by diluting or magnifying the drug's effect; whether or not its use will be permanent; if it can be obtained from natural sources; whether or not a generic substitute can be used and, if so, does the generic have the same potency, quality control and half-life. You owe it to yourself to ask questions about any foreign substance introduced into your system. At the very least, find out what is stated about your drug in a publication entitled "Prescription Drug Handbook" available from the American Association of Retired Persons (AARP) by calling 1-800-333-5600, or by consulting a book in your doctor's office titled "Physician's Desk Reference," an encyclopedia of drugs and medications. Your responsibility is to become informed about what others have prescribed for your health.

It is also your responsibility to reduce stroke risk factors which are within your power to control. Being overweight is risky. Reduce your intake of food. Even if your weight is satisfactory, go on a diet—a diet of nutritious foods. Add a generous helping of exercise. Lowering the intake of fat and sodium (salt) while increasing exercise may help reduce other risks such as high cholesterol, high blood pressure, and diabetes.

Smoking and drinking are very risky because they cause severe damage to the vascular system. For those who have already had a stroke, the best advice is to give up smoking and alcohol entirely. Such advice is easier said than done, since some claim tobacco and liquor can be as addictive as heroin. A number of our members continued to smoke, then suffered another stroke. One or two continued the habit after the second stroke, but died with the third. How tragic to have a harmful addiction stronger than the will to live.

Stroke: An Owner's Manual

♥

Chapter **8**

SERVE YOURSELF A GENEROUS HELPING OF HEALTH

Tips on overcoming the effects of a stroke.

♥

Chapter 8

SERVE YOURSELF A GENEROUS HELPING OF HEALTH

The best medicine is the lifestyle you prescribe for yourself.

H al was an engineer who pushed himself too hard at work in order to avoid the additional stress of a marriage which was falling apart. The resultant stroke he suffered was severely debilitating. His speech center was so badly disturbed it appeared he would never talk again; his right hand and leg were completely paralyzed. He barely had the strength to move along in a wheelchair. Years later, though one hand remained useless, an ankle brace was all he needed to help him walk. He began to recover some speech after a therapist used the technique of having him sing his name. (Singing and cursing are forms of automatic speech). As part of rehabilitation therapy, Hal became skillful in metalcraft. He began to teach a course in the craft to elementary school children, making the most use of one hand and a few words, "watch, try, good, beautiful." For the last five years there's been a waiting list for all six classes this reborn man teaches. The children aren't merely his students; they are the new love in his life.

In spite of a stroke which made speaking difficult and weakened his right side limbs, Joel refused to give up on two dreams. He wanted to return to architectural work, and to take an active part in his daughter's wedding. He was determined to walk her down the aisle and recite a blessing to the couple. Because he could no longer do fine drawing, he went to night school to study the new field of computer architecture. The old firm put him back to work. He strengthened his voice and leg by taking minor roles in amateur theater productions of musicals. He not only walked down the aisle and pronounced a blessing, he danced at the wedding.

Les had been a strong contributor in the small family business. He handled the front office and repaired equipment when necessary. Though there was no evident damage, his type of stroke took away the ability to perform any of those duties. It also caused him painful self-doubt. Once he understood that he had actually lost the capacity to perform as before, he started to work around his disabilities. A couple years after the stroke, he turned to assisting those who suffered similar types of loss. He holds his head high today, strong in the knowledge he is able to make a substantial contribution to others.

Wes's left leg is weak and his left arm almost useless. He had been an avid golfer before the stroke. With some coaching and the use of specially made clubs, he got back on the golf course. After many hours of practice he regained much of his earlier skill. Now, he coaches others who have suffered motor loss. Recently he shot a 28 on a short nine-hole course. Most good golfers with healthy limbs would be proud to score as low as 36 on the same course.

Max was fortunate in escaping damage to his communication faculties, but the stroke sentenced him to a wheelchair. He set three goals for himself: get a master's degree in Public Relations, live on his own, lead as normal a life as possible. The first two have been accomplished and the third goal will be reached soon when he wheels down the aisle with his childhood sweetheart.

Every one of the support group members is a success story in some way. You can create your story, but there's no time for depression, self-pity, shame or isolation. For example, many stroke survivors hide their flaccid or clawed hand. During meetings we encourage placement of the involved hand out in the open, with the fingers worked on by the good hand. There are at least three healthy reasons for this: movement of the fingers is beneficial therapy, a raised hand assists circulation, and hiding the hand is a sign of shame. There are other things within your power to do which will aid in your recovery.

BE SOCIAL

Even though some of the old friends may not come around as before, keep in mind that there may be several reasons for their staying away. Few people understand strokes. They are uncomfortable with someone who may have difficulty communicating as before. Many people avoid loved ones because they can't stand to witness the other person's pain. In general, people have difficulty dealing with those who are ill.

Phil had a wife and three children when he was struck down. None of them could tolerate living with a speechless, bedridden stranger. His wife, unable to stay with him "in sickness and health," got a divorce. The children stayed away. About ten years later, one of the sons, filled with shame and remorse, arrived at the doorstep of his father's new family home. Phil walked to the door to embrace his son and, with the wisdom gained conquering his stroke, softly told the tearful young man, "I love you. I understand."

SLOW DOWN

I cannot emphasize enough that you must slow down. Learn to be patient with yourself. Regardless of the degree of injury suffered, all stroke survivors have had one hell-of-a kick in the head, the center of the nervous system. Years of slow, steady recovery face you. As stated earlier, don't expect to perform anything with either the speed or accuracy once enjoyed. If you were always on the go before, the stroke will force you to learn a new talent known as taking it slow and easy.

USE EXTRA CARE

Those fortunate enough to return to driving must change old habits. If you were a cautious driver before, become more cautious. Give yourself extra time to get wherever you're going ... then take the extra time. Few stroke survivors ought to use the freeways, no matter how confident they feel. Freeways are a risky enterprise even for those in the best of health. They certainly aren't the place to drive for anyone with the slightest impairment.

Actions once performed automatically now require close attention. A commonly related experience is that of backing down a ladder, starting to lose balance and being unable to recover in time to prevent a jarring fall.

At times even the simple act of walking requires caution. When stroke survivors get tired they bump against door jambs or have trouble navigating around furniture. It's all part of the injury you have received. Listen to your body. It may be telling you to get more rest.

BE INDEPENDENT

In spite of all these cautions, don't be afraid to be independent. The battle against stroke is won the day a stroke survivor says, "I have some disabilities, but I'm not handicapped." It's the realization that he's different but not at a disadvantage. In truth, he's ahead of the game by having survived the most devastating of illnesses and moved on with life.

Fred understands everything, but can speak only a few words. He navigates in a wheelchair moved by his one good hand. He has his own apartment where he cooks and cleans for himself. He loves to travel, preferably with a lady friend. But being without a traveling companion has never held him back. As best he can, he makes the trip arrangements, gets to the airport, enjoys the flight, sees the sights and makes it back home. The "best he can" is equal to the task.

GET INVOLVED

If you had a hobby before, don't be afraid to try it again. Joe, an artist, had to switch hands, but his work hasn't suffered. Sid was able to return to his favorite fishing holes when he substituted tackle specially designed for one-handed use. Ted can't speak, but has no motor loss. Though he will always mourn the loss of a voice, it hasn't prevented him from returning to the golf game he loves and has mastered. Dan's communication is intact, but his left hand and leg are badly impaired. Special tools have made it possible for him to garden from his wheelchair using one hand. Several of the group have become self-appointed caregivers. They keep track of each person, help those who need help, visit those who are lonely and pay special attention to getting new members started on the path to recovery. For them it's a full time, fulfilling activity.

The best medicine is the lifestyle you prescribe for yourself.

♥

Chapter **9**

SOME THINGS REQUIRE
SPECIAL INSTRUCTION

Falling, getting up, driving.

Stroke: An Owner's Manual

Chapter 9

SOME THINGS REQUIRE SPECIAL INSTRUCTION

To paraphrase from Proverbs, "Let your pride and haughty spirit go before a fall and further destruction."

I t's easy for a stroke survivor to fall, but hard to fall correctly. Getting up may also be quite difficult. Each requires expert schooling. You need to be taught how to twist during a fall in order to reduce the impact on your body.

Getting up requires a good deal of maneuvering so that the strong limbs do all the work. Sometimes a cane is all that is needed for the support necessary to rise to a steady standing position. Sometimes it's necessary to crawl to a chair or other firmly planted object. Instruction is required to learn the various alternative methods of rising safely. (A simple way for healthy people to get a small taste of what it feels like to have a motor loss is to attempt to rise from a prone position using only one arm and leg. Good luck!)

To paraphrase from Proverbs, "Let your pride and

haughty spirit go before a fall and further destruction."

Most stroke survivors long for the day they can get behind the wheel of a car. Few other activities provide injured people with such a sense of freedom and independence as driving. However, what formerly was done almost automatically, actually demands physical capabilities which are often disrupted by a stroke. For example, the nerves for sight follow paths which circle the entire brain. Strokes often damage these nerves, causing losses ranging from mere neglect of a portion of the field of vision to complete blindness. It is possible to adapt cars so they can be driven by people who are limited in the use of their limbs and who have partial vision. But the capacity to drive is severely reduced when aphasia causes the language of road signs to be incomprehensible.

There are schools which specialize in teaching driving to the disabled. As soon as you feel eager to give it a try, have a teacher at one of those schools evaluate your chances of getting back on the road. And happy motoring!

♥

Chapter **10**

ONE PICTURE IS WORTH A THOUSAND WORDS

Communication without words.

♥

Chapter **10**

ONE PICTURE IS WORTH A THOUSAND WORDS

We believe in the theory that words make up only a small percentage of the means of communication.

Our insensitive world considers communication by speech to be such a measure of intelligence that the word for stupid (dumb) and the word for being unable to speak are the same. Often, out of ignorance, close friends or family members avoid the company of stroke survivors who have aphasia. How terrible it must be for those whose voices have been silenced to be subjected to the further pain of social isolation.

Many stroke survivors are able to speak, but the words may come out very slowly or be almost unintelligible. Imagine what it must be like to have clear thoughts in your head which sound to others like gibberish when you attempt to express them. How terrifying to have strangers back away or point as if dealing with an animal. For someone who was able to speak at one time, the sudden loss of ability to communicate verbally must be like dying a little each day. Though it takes almost superhuman bravery to survive such an ordeal, there are many survivors among us.

Max knew after several years of therapy that his only words would be a handful of automatic vulgarisms. He is able to write and draw, however, and he gets a few thoughts across with pencil and paper. Interestingly, one of the oft heard comments in our group is, "Won't someone shut Max up so the rest of us get a chance to talk." He has memorized over a hundred expressions in Indian sign language. The signing plus the meaning he conveys with facial expressions, and pictures provide him with a good sized vocabulary and, quite often, more meaningful communication than those who are long-winded. Significantly, what he lacks in sound he makes up for in sensitivity. Max is always the first to notice if another is feeling blue. He's always the first to communicate love and concern. Dumb? Like a fox he is.

Several others in the group are unable to verbalize. One would expect silence to be a dreadful sentence. Nevertheless, were a stranger to enter our midst, his best chance to pick out the speechless would be to locate those who gesture, draw or write a great deal, send messages with their facial expressions, laugh and smile the most.

We believe in the theory that words make up only a small percentage of the means of communication.

And we see the theory in action every time we meet.

♥

Chapter **11**

STRESS CAN BE VERY STRESSFUL

A major stroke risk factor.

Chapter 11

STRESS CAN BE VERY STRESSFUL

None of us has the power to change our family history, the aging process, or a condition of diabetes, but chronic stress is one of the several stroke risks we have a chance to control. For the sake of their very lives, it is imperative that stroke survivors reduce stress and learn how to "keep their cool."

S am says he knows why he had his stroke. Oblivious to those about him, he pushed hard at his job day and night striving to be the top man in his field. Part of the push was fueled by a ten-cigar-a-day smoking habit. An artery finally broke down under the stress. One of his stock-in-trade quips is that he has a fifty-three year old stroke. The same drive which probably made him ill was applied to healing. Today, a stranger meeting Sam would never know he had been without speech for many months and was paralyzed. Sam still has a powerful will to succeed but his goals have changed. As no other before him in our group, he strives to help those who are hurt, lonely or bewildered. Whatever stress he may feel being a sensitive care-giver is undoubtedly the healthy variety because he has become a stronger and finer man.

Mal was a litigator for a large law firm. Day after day he was under the constant pressure of battling an adversary from another firm, one whom he one day would have to face in the tense arena of a court. The constant pressure took its toll in an ever heightening blood pressure, increased heart rate, added cholesterol and production of chemicals in his blood damaging to the vascular system. His arteries were in a chronic pressure-cooker destined to explode. When he was passed over for promotion in favor of a younger man, something gave way in the left hemisphere of his brain. He may never again string words together with ease, much less argue a legal position. However, he and his wife have turned adversity into sweetness. They retired to an area where soft blue skies look down upon them as they engage in the kindly stress of making their way around a golf course.

A brilliant internist known for his personal dedication to patients got so emotionally involved with several difficult cases the stress caused a major artery in his cerebellum to go into spasm. Ordinarily, instant death would follow from the large loss of blood supply to the brain resulting from such a spasm. He survived but not without damage to that area of his brain. Threat of a reoccurrence forced him into retirement. Typical of the results of damage in the rear brain, he is left with an unsteady gait and uncertain balance. He talks with a twinkle in his eye of how he tends to roll head over heels whenever he bends to tie a shoelace. He says the acrobatics are a small price to pay for survival.

It has been proven medically that chronic stress exacerbates other well-established causes of strokes. This harmful stress can increase blood pressure, raise the level of blood cholesterol, increase the heart beat rate, and cause certain chemicals to be produced in the body which harm the arterial system.

None of us has the power to change our family history, the aging process, or a condition of diabetes, but chronic stress is one of the several stroke risks we have a chance to control. These are times when too much stress seems to have left much of our society with skins too thin to hold back inner turmoil. We hear it in obscenities shouted by motorists; we see it in the degree to which rudeness has replaced courtesy in our day to day activities. For the sake of their very lives, it is imperative that stroke survivors reduce stress and learn how to "keep their cool."

♥

Chapter **12**

SUPPORT GROUPS ARE A MUST

How groups help stroke survivors and
family survivors.

♥

Chapter **12**

SUPPORT GROUPS ARE A MUST

Rather than "misery loves company," the effect is one of "company softens misery." I have seen the uncaring become sensitive; the ambitious, satisfied; the nervous, relaxed; the ignorant, educated; the weak, strong; the unloved, fulfilled.

I t is incomprehensible to me how anyone can overcome the psychological set-back of a damaging stroke without the help of a stroke support group. The group approach is similar in a way to that used in psychiatry, the essential differences being that the stroke group is conducted by a facilitator, and several of the members may be totally incapable of verbal communication. Some theorists maintain that support groups should be limited to ten members, physically arranged in a circle small enough so that each can touch his neighbor. However, while it adheres to the theory of being in a circular configuration, the most successful group I participate in has at least fifteen regularly in attendance, and often as many as twenty-five.

Typically, a trained "facilitator" moves the discussion along, encouraging each participant to reveal his problems, concerns or successes. Since there is a commonality of experience which stroke survivors share, such discussions rapidly involve the entire group. Those without speech find ways to communicate; those whose words are labored find an audience of infinite patience; those who have difficulty with meaning find helpful encouragement; those with paralysis or paresthesia are with others similarly injured. Before long, members discard their self-consciousness at the doorway. They find none of the unfriendliness encountered in the outside world where the healthy ones often shun those who have difficulty communicating or appear to be disfigured.

Many who enter the circle for the first time are unable to hold back tears. They find comfort in learning others faced the same problem. Rather than "misery loves company," the effect is one of "company softens misery." Tears become understood rather than undermining, especially when the crying of new members prompts reddened eyes among the old-timers.

New members usually arrive burdened with symptoms of fear, depression, selfishness, anger, loneliness and bewilderment. In the healing process groups can provide, not only are these symptoms alleviated but most participants grow in ways never contemplated during their healthy lives. I have seen the uncaring become sensitive; the ambitious, satisfied; the nervous, relaxed; the ignorant, educated; the weak, strong; the unloved, fulfilled.

Though not intended as a substitute for personal research, the cumulative knowledge about strokes within a support group may surpass that of some health practitioners, even ones who work in the field. Regular discussion topics in the large group referred to in paragraph one of this chapter include the physiology, causation and prevention of strokes. Members stay apprised of the latest advances described in medical journals, or receive information through lecture programs presented by practitioners in related fields.

As indicated earlier, family members need support groups as much if not more than the survivors. It doesn't take long to realize that more than one person is the "victim" of a stroke. In the case of a wife who has been dependent on her spouse for earnings and the management of financial affairs, there may be a more severe wrenching out of the normal pattern of life than that for the one whose brain is injured. Not only is she faced with the responsibility of the family's economic survival, she must learn to be a constant nurse. No greater test of the strength of a relationship can be imagined than that of a stroke survivor and spouse. The disruption of a household is just as common when the wife is the one who has the stroke.

About fifteen years ago, Beth was hit not by one but by two strokes which wiped out her voice and left her totally paralyzed. Her husband gave up his medical practice to become her constant nurse. The running of house and home became new responsibilities for which he was ill prepared. Several years passed before she had gained enough speech and physical strength to relieve him of some of the day to day household chores. Throughout the many months of caring for his wife, he needed not only the moral support of wives whose husbands had suffered strokes, he also had to have their advice about being a house-husband. At the same time that he was receiving support from the spousal group, she became actively involved with a support group of stroke survivors. The two literally were able to survive their ordeal because of the advice and support received from others. To this very day, they remain involved with both groups out of gratitude for the help they received and in the hope of being of service to others who may be similarly hurt. Beth and her husband are an extreme example of a couple's mutual need for group support due to a devastating speech and movement loss.

Surprisingly, however, the greatest value of support groups may come when the stroke damage is least noticeable. Those who suffer right hemisphere strokes may show no obvious signs of communication or motor loss yet have the utmost need for knowledge, acceptance and understanding. Precisely because the damage cannot be observed, this type of stroke probably destroys more close relationships than others. How long could you go on living with someone who misinterprets innocent remarks, misreads facial expressions, acts like a fool in public, talks everyone's ear off, constantly gets confused by physical surroundings, can't keep track of finances, becomes instantly angry with small provocation, can't put two and two together, is insensitive to others needs, overestimates abilities, fails to recognize short-comings, or talks forever without coming to the point?

Malory's wife wasn't able to handle changes in his personality for more than a few months before she sued for divorce. He himself wasn't aware of the damage inflicted upon him by the stroke until others in the group convinced him they had gone through the same experience.

Dick and his wife stayed together because the facilitator arranged for an early meeting with a stroke survivor who explained to them the hell to which he had subjected his own wife. Being forewarned helped them over the roughest hurdles.

Maury's right hemisphere stroke not only caused a number of the subtle behavioral changes noted above but included paralysis of the left hand and weakened left leg. He and his wife needed all the education a group could impart. Not only was she required to take control over their lives and become a part-time nurse, she had to withstand his obnoxious behavior. He needed to understand his losses and learn how to control his emotions as quickly as possible or he was sure to lose her. Equipped with understanding, they were able to start hand in hand down an extremely rough road toward accommodation.

Ralph, a right hemisphere stroke survivor, entered the circle carrying the terrible burden of having lost his business acumen, not having any understanding of what had happened to him, but feeling great anger "over the whole damn thing." He talked forever about what he believed he could accomplish and his puzzlement over constant failure. Suggestions from group members were misunderstood. His usual response to advice was anger. But he was dealing with knowledgeable people who understood what was wrong. After many months, he began to accept the fact that brain cells had died, taking with them controls he once had. In time he has come to understand the need to "work around" what no longer exists, to discover his strengths and capitalize on them. With understanding, Ralph demonstrates a lessening of anger. He recognizes the need to abandon old unrealistic expectations and start a new direction in his life. Recently, he took on the job of assisting a stroke survivor who lost all mobility. Success with his new friend has made the worry lines in Ralph's face disappear.

Ted kept his physical strength but was deprived of all words except a few numbers and the usual vulgarities. He became severely depressed when he realized further speech therapy would not increase his verbalizing beyond the repetitious use of "four-five, four-five" whenever he wanted to express himself. (Some aphasia survivors are left with little more than one or two sounds whenever they try to speak. Bill is only able to say "Te dat, te dat") Several in the group got Ted back to playing the game of golf he once loved. It took a great deal of time for him to grasp what happened and to accept the fact his speech will never improve significantly. With the acceptance there came a form of resignation. Soon he could communicate his feelings to the group through body language: expression in the face, hands and posture. One of the best group healing tools is humor. When the members are able to joke about their losses, they're well on their way to health. During one session, without realizing it Ted added the number six to his usual "four five." Another member walked over, shook his hand and congratulated him on having increased his vocabulary by one third. There was a brief moment of suspense, then a burst of laughter from Ted followed by the entire group. The healing had begun.

Although the length of time spent in a group varies, each of the members finally is ready to graduate, sufficiently fortified to face the years ahead on his own two feet, with or without a cane or wheelchair. He will have seen numerous types of strokes, become expert in ways to reduce or eliminate his personal risks of suffering another, learned ways to maintain good health, gained life-long friendships, and, most important of all, been started on the path to a sense of self-worth.

Finding a stroke support group or club merely requires contacting any one of a number of sources. On a national level, these include the American Heart Association at 7320 Greenville Avenue, Dallas, Texas 75231, (214) 373-6300; or the Courage Stroke Network at 3915 Golden Valley Road, Golden Valley, Minnesota 55422, toll free 1-800-553-6321; or the National Stroke Association at 300 East Hampden Ave., Suite 240, Englewood, Colorado 80110-2622, toll free 1-800-787-6537. Sponsors of other stroke support groups include the Easter Seal Society, rehabilitation facilities, visiting nurse associations and hospitals.

Perhaps the first support group in our country primarily concerned with providing fellowship, knowledge and understanding originated in the Speech Pathology Department of the Veterans Administration Center located in Long Beach, California. It began with a speech pathologist as facilitator and continues under the same arrangement. If the visitors it receives from foreign countries and from cities all over the United States are a measure of success, it has no peer anywhere in the world.

Another type of group of great value is an activity center. Activity centers are concerned more with "doing" than "healing," although the two go hand in hand. At such centers stroke survivors are able to spend the better part of a day participating in activities ranging from card playing and crafts to mere socializing. For many spouses, such centers are a godsend, providing them the only free time they get during a week. Some groups take trips as short as a bus ride to a local art museum, as long as an overseas tour. The obvious benefit of doing such things is the replanting of normalcy in a life yanked out of its roots. Non "social" card players might envy the silent seriousness of a game where players signal rather than gossip or bicker. Though there is the unhappy trade-off due to the need for a wooden rack to replace the hand which can't hold a hand, nobody's complaining.

♥

Chapter **13**

THE TREES AND THE FOREST

Seeing change take place.

♥

Chapter **13**

THE TREES AND THE FOREST

Progress often is best measured by those who themselves have been similarly hurt. They are well aware of the fine tuning which never ceases within the amazing instrument of the brain.

Earlier references have been made to the fact that certain aspects of the condition of a stroke survivor will continue getting better so long as he works at it. Any improvement which occurs after several years have passed may be so small, however, that he or those in daily contact with him observe no change. It's the old saw about not seeing the forest for the trees. Progress often is best measured by those who themselves have been similarly hurt. They are well aware of the fine tuning which never ceases within the amazing instrument of the brain.

The Les we first knew was deeply depressed, used gestures to indicate a desire for suicide, refused to take charge of his health needs and constantly berated himself. Several of the more forceful group members set out to steer him into a more positive mode. Week after week they gave him supportive encouragement, working on his self-image, battling his cigarette habit, not permitting him to feel sorry about his useless right arm or lack of speech. In time, especially after being introduced to one-armed golf which he quickly mastered, he began to appreciate the half full portion of what fate had served him. Within two years he had made a complete turnabout. Today he is one of the hardest working caregivers in the group, spreading the joy of life to other newcomers with a hearty left handshake. Though the words are labored, he talks about how important it is to enjoy life. He has lost weight, has a full heart and an empty cigarette pocket. Everything has improved except his memory of the Les we first knew. He feels such joy now, he finds it inconceivable that he ever was in such a negative frame of mind.

Willy was an engineer responsible for quality assurance. Though he could still move his right arm and hand following the stroke, they were cocked at an odd angle and had little dexterity. He could speak, but the sentences often were disjointed, the words somewhat slurred. With a downturned mouth he constantly used the word "can't" when referring to his condition. That particular word raises the ire of many who "couldn't" at one time but fought hard enough to substitute "can do" for "can't." As Willy's physical strength returned, the down lines in his face took a pushing around from the others until his smile returned. Physiotherapy brought some significant gains in his right side movements, and he was on his way. Now, when referring to his speech difficulties, he says, "Not as good as before," instead of "can't talk," and he proudly demonstrates his improved arm and hand agility. We well remember the man who felt his life no longer had any quality, but he denies that person ever existed.

Ted was in a forest of trouble a few years ago. Not only had the stroke severed the line of communication from thought to verbalization, but he seemed unable to comprehend the speech of others. It often was necessary to wave and get his attention so he would focus on the person speaking. Even when focused, he had the distant look of one who is lost. Over many months, his aspect changed. We would watch his eyes move from speaker to speaker, notice the changes in expression which indicated he was following some of the discussions. Since he never lost reading comprehension, a few notes on a blackboard always were of special benefit to him, as they still are today. But the change is remarkable. No longer is he totally out of the communication loop. His face is relaxed, his manner easy and his smile infectious. Moments of moodiness still haunt him on occasion, but he soon is smiling again. Someone observing Ted for the first time might only notice those limitations which he still deeply regrets... few words and the need for occasional assistance to help him understand those who speak too fast. Nevertheless, the improvement in spirit and self acceptance described above continue day by day.

Now, when we speak of the early dark days, his usual response is well within his communication capability, a four letter word accompanied by a look of denial. He has come out from behind the trees.

♥

Chapter **14**

BRAVERY IN THE FACE OF IGNORANCE

Daytime nightmares.
Carrying on in a world unfamiliar with
the effects of stroke.

Stroke: An Owner's Manual

♥

Chapter **14**

BRAVERY IN THE FACE OF IGNORANCE

Those who are cruelly damaged by stroke are hard pressed not to die a little each day when they are constantly confronted by a world that is almost totally ignorant of the effects of a stroke.

In The World According to Garp, John Irving ends his book with the words, "we are all terminal." He probably has in mind the one event, birth, which eventually leads to the death of each of us. Today, however, the word terminal is more commonly used when referring to an incurable illness which renders our days numbered and frequently painful. For those coping with such terminal conditions, the word "courage" immediately springs to mind. People who survive heart attacks are frequently in a second category, able to get on with their lives with a minimum of medical intervention and some fine-tuning of life style. For heart attack survivors able to escape lingering disability through such small adjustments, the words "sensible" and "lucky" are applicable. But what about those who are cruelly damaged by stroke? Those with aphasia (disturbance in the communication center of the brain) to a severe degree are sentenced to live with little chance of being restored to their former selves, no matter how great the effort. Others with aphasia but still able to communicate in limited ways are hard pressed not to die a little each day when they are constantly confronted by a world that is almost totally ignorant of the effects of a stroke. The Queen in Alice in Wonderland could have been advising these stroke survivors when she said, "It takes all the running you can do to keep in the same place." For this latter group, the word "bravery" seems most applicable. Healthy people ordinarily get through a routine day without peril. For many disabled people, getting through any day is a tough workout. Moreover for those disabled by stroke, trying to do routine things may not only be difficult but terrifying. Perhaps what distinguishes a great many stroke survivors from those disabled by other causes is that the lightening bolt of stroke usually is two-pronged, striking both movement and language. The four-legged cane or two-wheeled chair can provide mobility for a damaged body. What vehicle does one use to "get around" when one's voice or comprehension is severely limited?

Several activities are hereby described in detail to illustrate how simple every-day matters can be especially trying for those who have both aphasia and physical disabilities. For each activity presented, a successful solution has been found and described by a real life stroke survivor.

BUSES

The simple matter of using public transportation can be very stressful for anyone with physical disabilities. High boarding steps and single handrails are the first challenges to be overcome. Physical stress can rise to trauma if that same person has aphasia. A possible scenario might find a stroke survivor trying to produce the correct fare with one good hand while balancing on one good leg and being unable to rely on words if any difficulty occurs. Getting aboard and paying are immediately followed by the fear (well founded) that the vehicle will start moving before a seat is secured. Parting may involve more apprehension because, again, there are high steps to negotiate, often with the simultaneous need to pull or push some door apparatus.

Adding another common problem to this mix results in a nightmarish brew. People with good language skills find it difficult to read street signs that pass swiftly by when viewed from a bus window. On whom is someone with aphasia to turn for assistance when it's time to get off the bus? The busy driver who is handed a prepared note? Maybe. A fellow passenger to whom a note can be offered? Perhaps.

Jack, who stopped driving as soon as he began having seizures, cannot read, has labored speech, one useless arm and a weak leg. But he is fortunate to have a determined fighting spirit. Like a lonely matador, he confronts the beastly bus and wins. He gets to the bus stop early enough to board ahead of others, and then relies on his good arm to hoist him up. As he pays with a pre-purchased pass, he hands the driver a typed note indicating his destination. Being first aboard usually gives him time to get seated while the rest of the passengers enter and pay. He has not only timed the trip but familiarized himself with landmarks near his street exit. He positions himself so he is able to tap the driver as a reminder that his destination is approaching. A second (but less desirable) alternative is to sit close to the rear door, and as the stop approaches, repeatedly signal until the bus driver takes note of him.

(Is it any wonder that being able to drive is so important to a stroke survivor's sense of independence and social integration?)

RESTAURANTS

Buses are duck soup compared to eating out. Almost all of our language and symbolic skill is called upon to order food, check the tab, calculate a tip, and then count the money. A language deficiency or inability to comprehend numbers would make these required steps almost impossible without assistance from a companion. Added physical problems (i.e., the use of only one hand, difficulty grasping and releasing utensils and glasses, the likelihood of choking on liquids or food) certainly would seem to take all flavor out of eating in public.

Rick, who can't stand his own cooking, uses a creative approach to make his frequent use of restaurants more pleasurable. He carries a pouch containing a set of special utensils (a "rocker" knife especially built to cut foods with one hand by use of a rocking motion and a "hands-off" drinking cup with a hospital type adjustable straw). The waiter is shown a printed card which lists Rick's limitations and ends with the words, "Your help will be greatly appreciated." Rick says he's occasionally been served a poor meal, but he's never felt uncomfortable or had poor service when he uses this strategy.

SUPER-MARKETS

Shopping in a large store usually begins with the challenge of mobilizing the strength to yank a metal basket free from the embrace of other baskets. The venture continues with the game of "dodge'em" as one heads down the aisles. Assuming one has the physical agility to steer around impasses, there are many other physical demands. A common problem for stroke survivors is a lack of hand strength or steadiness when grasping objects. Carefully balanced cans and jars must be avoided at the risk of creating a trail of fallen merchandise. Plastic bags at the fruit and vegetable counters are frustrating to open even for those with nimble fingers - - almost impossible for others. But if one is able to select merchandise without incident, the last and most difficult part of the journey must be faced: the checkout counter. On busy days one must go through a frenzy of stacking merchandise, trying to keep an eye on the totals coming from a checker's flying fingers, getting the requested amount of money paid quickly, searching for the place where the change comes clanging, and getting out of the way of the next person in line.

Bill, who loves to shop, avoids the crowd by selecting

a quiet time of a mid-week day to do his shopping. Though he has fair hand strength, he sticks to shelf food in plastic containers. He comes equipped with his own reusable cloth bags for fruit or vegetables. At the checkstand he tries to select a person who appears to have a pleasant manner and, when his turn arrives, he immediately tells the checker that he has difficulty with speech and movement. Most employees respond to him with extra courteous treatment, and box-boys almost always offer to help Bill load his car.

At stroke support meetings, members discuss techniques which may help to resolve problems associated with the day to day nightmares of life. It's the simple little things that are so hellish: the struggle to get caps on or off a toothpaste tube, switching in frustration to a push-button dispenser, the lava flow of paste ejected when a disobedient finger pushes too hard; reaching for a light switch but being unable to coordinate the movements required to grasp or move it; picking up a chicken leg and having the arm go into spasm as the food is raised to the mouth, and being unable to let go; the complete avoidance of using the telephone for fear of not being understood.

On rare occasions, they tell of hell itself. In Fred's case, his stroke caused him to have a brush with obscurity while in the very hands of those one would expect to be the most knowledgeable.

Following a stroke, Fred was discovered behind the wheel of his car unable to utter a word and in what appeared to be a catatonic state. His identification indicated he was entitled to treatment at a Veteran's Medical Center. While being treated there, he recovered physical movement but remained mute. In accordance with hospital procedure in such cases, the psychiatric department evaluated him. When unable to answer simple questions about his name, the date and the name of the president, they declared him incompetent. A local judge appointed an attorney to be his conservator (a type of guardian) to take possession of his property and dispose of it as deemed best for the man. Fortunately, Fred's path crossed that of a discerning speech pathologist who realized that the stroke had merely caused him to lose his speech. The word "merely" is used because Fred was about to be shunted off to an area of the hospital where he would have lived in virtual obscurity, cared for but forgotten. Today, through speech therapy, he has regained substantially all of his voice and all of his former independence.

Hopefully, the day will come when stroke and the nightmare it can cause will be common knowledge. Until then, the wounded have to be doubly brave ... brave enough not only to bear great loss but to carry on in a world without understanding.

♥

Chapter **15**

STROKES ARE NON-SEXIST

Women have as much pain and courage as men.

♥

Chapter 15

STROKES ARE NON-SEXIST

Women face the same all-consuming fight to restore health, dignity and self-esteem.

Although women are less at risk for stroke than men until later in life and generally recover from speech deficits somewhat easier, they nonetheless face the same all-consuming fight to restore health, dignity and self-esteem.

Picture this dramatic, dynamic real-life scene. It takes place at a stroke activity center sponsored by the American Heart Association, where a "mixed pairs" game of bridge exemplifies how strokes affect both sexes equally. Like the "crap game" made famous in GUYS AND DOLLS, this is one of the longest continuous bridge games in the world. It began with the opening of the center in 1978 and is played on Wednesday and Friday each week. Henry sits North. His speech is fine, but his left hand is useless. He places his cards on a wooden rack, somewhat similar to the kind used in a game of Scrabble, playing them with his good hand. Ellie, sitting South, has no problem with movement, but her speech is severely impaired. She bids by pointing to a diagram of the four suits then holding up fingers. She can also point to the word "pass," "double," or "redouble." Margie, unable to move either hand, sits West with her husband Lou at her side. Lou holds her hand and plays whatever card she asks for. Norm sits East. He, too, uses a rack to hold his cards because his right hand is severely uncoordinated; but unlike Henry, Norm's speech is slow, labored and slurred. Watching the action, one can't help but notice the high degree of caring concern, understanding, patience and comraderie which distinguishes their game from the intense competition that is evident when able-bodied persons play bridge.

In addition to several other women stroke survivors mentioned earlier in this handbook, a few other examples stand out in my memory.

Elise attended a local stroke support group sponsored by the United Stroke Foundation. Once a respected head nurse in charge of an intensive care unit at one of our largest hospitals, she suffered a stroke so severe that it wiped out her speech for many months. After a great deal of therapy, the only apparent residual from her ordeal is a small degree of hesitancy when she talks. If you have ever known someone who was a past stutterer but learned how to overcome the vocal interruption by sliding into a difficult letter or choosing a different word, you have an idea of Elise's speech pattern. She gave up nursing because the stress was harmful to her, but when the support group facilitator retired, Elise was selected to take over that job. Today the stroke support group members have the rare opportunity of having a leader who is "one of them." For Elise, facilitating the discussions gives her a non-stressful chance to continue her healing craft.

Sally's husband was so successful in the contracting business, the two of them were said to have a net worth over thirty million dollars. An extremely harsh stroke left her with little speech, a clawed hand and an extremely weakened leg. Though physically very small, her determined effort to regain her powers is herculean. Within two years she discarded the wheelchair, using a helpful arm or a cane to steady her walking. Now, she can be seen with the cane hanging nonchalantly from her arm as she walks unassisted to visit nearby neighbors. As part of her tenacious battle to win herself back, she created a charitable foundation and insisted on chairing the semi-monthly meetings of the board of directors. Though she hasn't perfected the language of Robert's Rules of Order, the two hour meetings move along smoothly under her direction. Recently when fatigue set in after a long extended meeting and blocked her recall of the expression "All in favor say Aye," she simply looked about the table and said, "Well, how about it?". Much of her day is spent visiting a wide variety of organizations which have received generous donations from her foundation. In just a few short years she has turned her affliction around and risen to a position of self-esteem never dreamed of when she was merely a healthy millionaire.

Until a stroke played havoc with her memory and the

motion of her right hand when she was sixty-eight years old, Janet was the ever-present church organist, social pianist and violist in a semi-professional string quartet. After her stroke, Janet set herself the task of rekindling the memory of all the music that had been her second voice since childhood. Though the musical phrases slowly returned, her right hand fingers refused to obey commands. Janet had difficulty keeping the bow from sliding down the strings or maintaining any consistent finger pressure on the organ or piano keys. But she never gave up trying. Just recently, after over three years of commitment, she revealed to her stroke support group that her church wanted her back at the organ for an upcoming Sunday service. The group not only insisted she attempt to play, they filled the front row bench to give her additional support. She made it through the entire service. The group members then began to press for viola performances before each support group session. Shortly after her seventy-first birthday, Janet joined her old quartet to play in the final number of one of their programs. The same support group that had gone to church for her was the first to rise to give her a standing ovation.

♥

Chapter **16**

A WORD ABOUT WORDS TO THOSE WHO CARE

Suggestions about making communication easier.
Listening instead of talking.
Being honest and sensitive.

♥

Chapter **16**

A WORD ABOUT WORDS TO THOSE WHO CARE

Stroke survivors, especially those with distrubed language centers (aphasia), are more comfortable when there is only one sound to deal with at a time.

I f you are among the few who not only enjoy good health but are concerned about helping those who are not so fortunate, some advice will be helpful to make your dealing with a KNOWN stroke survivor easier for both of you. The word "known" is accented because right hemisphere damage is rarely obvious.

As detailed in Chapter 6, strokes in the right brain may cause serious changes which are so subtle they are considered mere behavioral quirks rather than symptoms of brain damage. Actions such as talking too much, being socially inappropriate, misunderstanding another's expression, or arriving at illogical conclusions from a set of facts may not be recognized as deficiencies unless they are accompanied by some obvious physical impairment.

The information which follows, though intended primarily to raise your awareness of those special communication problems caused by strokes, may also be applicable to others in poor health.

ONE VOICE IS A CHALLENGE,
TWO A DISASTER

People with uninjured brains often enjoy what is commonly referred to as "wallpaper sound,"—background music or voices. Perhaps the electronic sound fills a need for company when one is alone. Stroke survivors, however, especially those with disturbed language centers (aphasia), are more comfortable when there is only one sound to deal with at a time. Too much reception disturbs their concentration; even music may be a confusing distraction. At a stroke activity center, uninformed volunteer staffers try to lighten the atmosphere by turning up the volume on a jazz station. There is a universal sigh of relief when the radio is unplugged.

If music is a distraction, simultaneous voices can become a tower of babble. There is a cardinal rule in our stroke support meetings: NO SIDE CONVERSATIONS. When the rule is broken, chances are one of the violators has right hemisphere damage (inappropriate social behavior combined with uncontrolled talking). The surest way to invite instant chaos is to allow two right hemisphere stroke survivors to sit next to each other.

Those with unimpaired brains struggle to carry on a phone conversation when someone else talks to them. Most people either plug the free ear, sign the other person to be quiet, or stop the call. Picture yourself on the phone; give the caller a strange accent; make it an overseas line; now add static. That combination is a somewhat exaggerated picture of what stroke survivors might face when they try to understand one normal voice. Add that combination to the other ear and comprehension is almost impossible. The solution is simple. One voice at a time ... slowly ... and no loud jazz.

LISTEN ... LISTEN ... AND LISTEN SOME MORE

Listening when a stroke survivor talks takes a great deal of patience because he may be coping with one of several types of problems. The thought inside his head usually is clear and precise, but he may be unable to plan how to express it. Or, he may be able to do the planning, but the words won't come out as organized. Or, the words are able to come out as planned, but motor nerve damage causes the sound to be unintelligible. While this manual is not intended to be technical, some facts related to the physiology of speech are so amazing, they may help in explaining how a small motor injury can cause a huge speech disturbance.

When we verbalize, there are approximately FOURTEEN DIFFERENT SOUNDS PRODUCED EVERY SECOND. Over ONE HUNDRED DIFFERENT MUSCLES are controlled and coordinated during speech and each of those muscles is controlled by an average of over ONE HUNDRED MOTOR UNITS. Simple multiplication (100 x 100 x 14) results in an astounding 140,000 NEUROMUSCULAR EVENTS REQUIRED

FOR EACH SECOND OF SPEECH. Is it any wonder an injury to a portion of the brain controlling these muscles may result in garbled speech? The wonder is that any of us is able to form words clearly.

DON'T TALK ... LISTEN SOME MORE

When a person has difficulty expressing himself, the natural tendency is to try to help, either by finishing the phrase, or stating what the listener believes the speaker wants to say. That type of assistance may be well-intended, but when the speaker is a stroke survivor, each interruption inhibits his concentrated effort to get the words out. In fact, hearing your voice may result in confusion rather than help. Joe says he would rather not talk than have someone constantly finish his sentence. His rationale is that he works so hard to get everything organized in his head, he feels cheated when not given the chance to complete the thought. People who have had some form of brain injury are sorely in need of time: time to organize a thought, time to get another's attention, time to finish what is started. The most caring of listeners is someone who isn't in a hurry to hear.

BE HONEST

When a stroke survivor's words aren't clear, it does no good pretending to understand; in fact, such pretense is counter-productive. Those whose speech may be slurred or garbled due to interference with those 140,000 neuro-muscular events usually speak clearer when they slow down, but they need to be made aware that a listener is having difficulty understanding them. During stroke support meetings, we use a hand signal to warn a person to slow down, and we ask those who are unclear to repeat themselves. Those with right hemisphere lesions tend to talk too much and too fast. They need to have someone signal them to apply the brakes. The signal works with everyone except Clay who has a runaway, record-breaking rate of speech. In a few moments, he exhausts the muscular capacity of his tongue and mouth to keep up with his attempted word production. All verbalization becomes a blur of sound. As a device to make his speech more intelligible, therapists devised a built-in metronome. Clay taps a finger against his leg in a slow rhythm meant to regulate his rate of speech. Now instead of signaling him to slow down, we just make sure his brake has started tapping.

New members of the support group tend to shy away from speaking because of the risk of failure, but in time they realize that being corrected is therapeutic and constructive, not critical.

BE SENSITIVE

Self-esteem takes a beating when one is unable to talk or be understood. However, as time goes on, many voiceless stroke survivors find other ways of communicating. The ability to get a thought across to another without using words is a large building block in the reconstruction of a toppled ego. Another who substitutes his own voice for that of the stroke survivor is not performing an act of kindness; rather, talking for another is an unwitting hinderance to recovery. Mack's wife loves him very much and after twenty-five years of marriage, she is able to anticipate what he wants to say. During the support meetings which are held without spouses, he gets all the time he needs to express himself as best he can. That's our way of loving and supporting him. But when he is with his wife, she tries to relieve his frustration by speaking for him. He communicates when he is with us; he is silent when with her.

In a marvelously mad play by Larry Shue titled The Foreigner, a woman speaks very loudly to someone she believes cannot understand her. Perhaps sheer volume will aid the meaning to penetrate. Sadly, many people do the same thing with those who have some form of aphasia, as if the lost language capability can be corrected with a loud voice. Aphasia isn't a problem to be addressed by increasing decibels but rather by heightening sensitivity.

You may not cure a damaged language center in a stroke survivor by applying these recommendations, but making communication easier will lessen the pain.

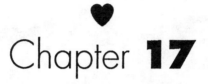

Chapter **17**

HELL OR REBIRTH?

New ways to measure success.

♥

Chapter **17**

HELL OR REBIRTH?

Refusal to give up is more than the beginning of recovery; it's halfway back. The trip ends with the pronouncement, "I'm disabled, but not handicapped."

Ask a man what he is and chances are he'll tell you what he does for a living. Rarely will a person answer the question with words such as, "I'm a sensitive human being who loves life," or "I'm a family man and a good friend," or "I'm a human being concerned about the fate of my fellow man," or "I'm one who respects the rights of others and works to secure those rights," or "I'm an individual trying to make some creative contribution to society." As bad luck would have it, most people define themselves only by reference to their occupations. It's worse luck when a stroke causes instant retirement. The "self" which was esteemed dies with the job title.

All of us are programmed to expect injuries to heal, given the proper care and treatment. Stroke survivors often tell of awaiting the day the paralysis or aphasia is gone. Even after years of living with the realization of permanent disability, many confess to the continued belief they will wake from the nightmare to find themselves whole. They dream of the morning when they can rise, go to work and be a person once again.

The illness follows a pattern. First the recognition something terrible has happened. Next the dread realization that neither you nor anyone else can repair the damage. This may be followed by the additional insult of dependency on others for mobility, or even more degrading, for assistance in the performance of simple necessary bodily functions. An independent adult becomes a dependent child in one stroke of horrible fate. Without help, many lack the strength to fight such dehumanization. They retreat to darkness, hiding from life until death brings relief. Too often, ignorant family members condemn loved ones to institutional hiding places without attempting a single probe to search for life, life in the form of an active mind behind the veil of a few dead brain cells.

But with help the fighters have a chance. Tens of thousands of them reject early burial. Refusal to give up is more than the beginning of recovery; it's halfway back. The trip ends with the pronouncement, "I'm disabled, but not handicapped." In our groups one after another readily admits to pre-stroke days of total self-involvement, lack of concern for others, the desire only to make it big, the belief that getting ahead was more important than having a heart. Then mortality rose up and hit them right in the brain.

Suddenly, the realization you have no control over your life makes the life you have a very precious thing.

All of the old methods you may have used to measure self-worth die along with the brain cells. They don't add up any more. It's time for new math. How have I helped myself to recover today? How can I contribute to the well-being of the guy next to me? What else can I do to make life more pleasant for my family or my community? Are there new challenges for me to conquer?

How you add up in answering those questions becomes the new "bottom line" of your value as a human being. Stroke survivors affirm life when they discover the pleasure of feeling loving concern for others. It begins and ends with survival. Start with making yours meaningful, then take on the world.

♥

Chapter **18**

RESOURCES

National and Regional Stroke Support Networks.

♥
Chapter **18**

RESOURCES

F inding a stroke support group or club may take little more than a couple of telephone calls. Listed below are several national and regional organizations which can lead you to groups close to your home. They can also make available to you additional literature about stroke or they can suggest sources to solve your specific problems.

NATIONAL

American Heart Association
7320 Greenville Avenue, Dallas, Texas 75231
(214) 373-6300

The Courage Stroke Network
3915 Golden Valley Road
Golden Valley, Minnesota 55422
Toll Free: 1-800-553-6321

The National Stroke Association
300 East Hampden Ave., Suite 240
Englewood, Colorado 80110-2654
Toll Free 1-800-787-6537

REGIONAL

Evergreen Stroke Association
9423 SE 36th Street
Mercer Island, WA 98040
206-461-7839

Nebraska Stroke Foundation
P.O. Box 67004
Lincoln, NE 68506
402-435-1698

Oregon Stroke Association
1015 NW 22nd Avenue
Portland, OR 97210
503-229-7124

Organization for After Stroke Resources
1150 N. Mountain Avenue, #208
Upland, CA 91786
714-985-0120

Residential Aphasia Program
University of Michigan
Communicative Disorders Clinic
1111 East Catherine
Ann Arbor, MI 48109
313-764-8440

Self-Help Clearinghouse
St. Clares-Riverside Medical Center
Pocono Road
Denville, NJ 07834
908-625-9565

Stroke Association of Kentucky
P.O. Box 4415
Lexington, KY 40544
606-233-5760

Stroke Association of Southern Califomia
522 South Sepulveda Boulevard, #101
Los Angeles, CA 90049
310-475-2714

Stroke Groups of Texas
12503 Mooredale Lane, B-19506
Houston, TX 77024
713-465-0943

Sponsors of other stroke support groups include the Easter Seal Society, rehabilitation facilities, visiting nurse associations and hospitals.

WHAT OTHERS ARE SAYING ABOUT THIS BOOK

"He expresses many of the problems which are common to stroke patients in a most eloquent and descriptive fashion. One important use of the manuscript would be to aid patients in making an adjustment and acceptance of stroke clubs. Acceptance of many of the sage comments in this manuscript might ease their transition back into society and help erase the shame, denial and reproach from which many stroke victims suffer."

Milton L. Fort, M.D., Co-Chief, Neuro Stroke Service
RANCHO LOS AMIGOS MEDICAL CENTER

"The author provides tips on continuing recovery and home management after formal rehab training, along with information about redeveloping skills. He covers the causes of stroke, degrees of improvement, personality changes, compensation for speech or motor loss, and coping mechanisms, documenting the information with real life success stories. MOST OF ALL HE OFFERS UNDERSTANDING, ENCOURAGEMENT AND HOPE TO THE FAMILIES AND TO THOSE STROKE SURVIVORS WHO ARE WILLING AND ABLE TO LEARN."

Mildred Selenkow, B.S., P.T., Baltimore, Maryland

"The material Mr. Josephs has written will be tremendously helpful not only for persons who have suffered a cerebrovascular accident (stroke), but it will also help their family members to better understand the changes which can occur on a cognitive, physical and social basis. Many of us in the health care profession do not do a good job in explaining what has happened, what can be expected and how to better deal with the residual effects of a stroke. This information will be invaluable."

H. Richard Adams, M.D.
(World Renowned Head-trauma Expert)
Chairman of the Professional Advisory Board,
Betty Clooney Foundation for Persons with Brain Damage

ORDER FORMS

YES! Please send **STROKE: AN OWNER'S MANUAL**

_____ copies at $14.95 each = $ _____

Shipping and handling $1.75 per book = $ _____

California residents add $1.23 sales tax per book = $ _____

Total = $ _____

☐ Please include information on quantity discounts.

Make check or money order payable to: AMADEUS PRESS-B
Send to: PO Box 13011 • Long Beach, CA 90803

I understand I may return the book for a full refund within 30 days of purchase if for any reason I'm not satisfied.

YES! Please send **STROKE: AN OWNER'S MANUAL**

_____ copies at $14.95 each = $ _____

Shipping and handling $1.75 per book = $ _____

California residents add $1.23 sales tax per book = $ _____

Total = $ _____

☐ Please include information on quantity discounts.

Make check or money order payable to: AMADEUS PRESS-B
Send to: PO Box 13011 • Long Beach, CA 90803

I understand I may return the book for a full refund within 30 days of purchase if for any reason I'm not satisfied.